Wrestling Training Log

INFORMATIONS

NAME

ADDRESS

E-MAIL ADDRESS

WEBSITE

PHONE **FAX**

EMERGENCY CONTACT PERSON

PHONE **FAX**

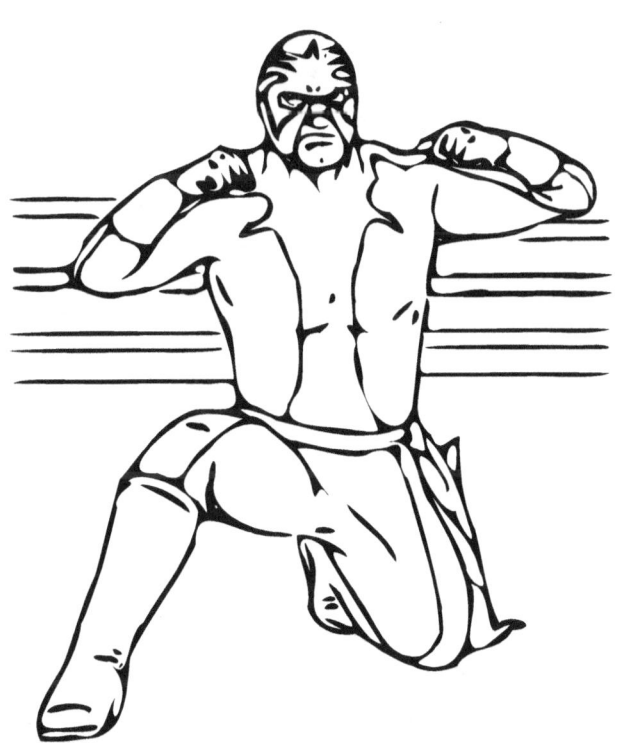

Dedication

This Wrestling Training Journal is dedicated to all the wrestlers out there who want to keep track of their training and document their findings in the process.

You are my inspiration for producing books and I'm honored to be a part of keeping all of your Wrestling notes and records organized.

This journal notebook will help you record your details about tracking your wrestling training.

Thoughtfully put together with these sections to record: Date & Time, Weeks, Hours Trained, Coach, Goals, Warm-up, Drills, Technique 1 & 2, & Notes.

How to Use this Book

The purpose of this book is to keep all of your Wrestling Training notes all in one place. It will help keep you organized.

This Wrestling Training Journal will allow you to accurately document every detail about your training sessions. It's a great way to chart your course through recording your trainings.

Here are examples of the prompts for you to fill in and write about your experience in this book:

1. Date & Time - Write the date and time.

2. Weeks - Record what week you're on.

3. Hours Trained - Log the number of hours you trained.

4. Coach - Write the name of your coach.

5. Goals - Record the goals you have set for yourself.

6. Warm-Up/ Drills - Log your warm up and drills you did.

7. Technique 1 & 2 - Write the techniques you worked on during this session.

8. Sure Notes - Blank lined space for recording any additional information you want to write or note, such as any nutrition goals, other player in your class notes, skills you need improving, your discipline strategy, daily, weekly & monthly goals, etc.

Wrestling Training Log

DATE **WEEKS** **HOURS TRAINED**
COACH **TIME**

GOALS

WARM UP / DRILLS

TECHNIQUE 1

TECHNIQUE 2

NOTES

Wrestling Training Log

DATE   **WEEKS**   **HOURS TRAINED**

COACH   **TIME**

GOALS

WARM UP / DRILLS

TECHNIQUE 1

TECHNIQUE 2

NOTES

Wrestling Training Log

DATE **WEEKS** **HOURS TRAINED**
COACH **TIME**

GOALS

WARM UP / DRILLS

TECHNIQUE 1

TECHNIQUE 2

NOTES

Wrestling Training Log

DATE WEEKS HOURS TRAINED
COACH TIME

GOALS

WARM UP / DRILLS

TECHNIQUE 1

TECHNIQUE 2

NOTES

Wrestling Training Log

DATE   **WEEKS**   **HOURS TRAINED**

COACH   **TIME**

GOALS

WARM UP / DRILLS

TECHNIQUE 1

TECHNIQUE 2

NOTES

....
....
....
....

Wrestling Training Log

DATE WEEKS HOURS TRAINED
COACH TIME

GOALS

WARM UP / DRILLS

TECHNIQUE 1

TECHNIQUE 2

NOTES

Wrestling Training Log

DATE   **WEEKS**   **HOURS TRAINED**

COACH   **TIME**

GOALS

WARM UP / DRILLS

TECHNIQUE 1

TECHNIQUE 2

NOTES

....
....
....
....

Wrestling Training Log

DATE _____   **WEEKS** _____   **HOURS TRAINED** _____

COACH _____   **TIME** _____

GOALS

WARM UP / DRILLS

TECHNIQUE 1

TECHNIQUE 2

NOTES

....
....
....
....

Wrestling Training Log

DATE   **WEEKS**   **HOURS TRAINED**

COACH   **TIME**

GOALS

WARM UP / DRILLS

TECHNIQUE 1

TECHNIQUE 2

NOTES

Wrestling Training Log

DATE   WEEKS   HOURS TRAINED
COACH   TIME

GOALS

WARM UP / DRILLS

TECHNIQUE 1

TECHNIQUE 2

NOTES

Wrestling Training Log

DATE **WEEKS** **HOURS TRAINED**
COACH **TIME**

GOALS

WARM UP / DRILLS

TECHNIQUE 1

TECHNIQUE 2

NOTES

....
....
....
....

Wrestling Training Log

DATE WEEKS HOURS TRAINED
COACH TIME

GOALS

WARM UP / DRILLS

TECHNIQUE 1

TECHNIQUE 2

NOTES

....
....
....
....

Wrestling Training Log

DATE **WEEKS** **HOURS TRAINED**
COACH **TIME**

GOALS

WARM UP / DRILLS

TECHNIQUE 1

TECHNIQUE 2

NOTES

Wrestling Training Log

DATE WEEKS HOURS TRAINED
COACH TIME

GOALS

WARM UP / DRILLS

TECHNIQUE 1

TECHNIQUE 2

NOTES

Wrestling Training Log

DATE **WEEKS** **HOURS TRAINED**

COACH **TIME**

GOALS

WARM UP / DRILLS

TECHNIQUE 1

TECHNIQUE 2

NOTES

....
....
....
....

Wrestling Training Log

DATE   **WEEKS**   **HOURS TRAINED**

COACH   **TIME**

GOALS

WARM UP / DRILLS

TECHNIQUE 1

TECHNIQUE 2

NOTES

....
....
....
....

Wrestling Training Log

DATE **WEEKS** **HOURS TRAINED**
COACH **TIME**

GOALS

WARM UP / DRILLS

TECHNIQUE 1

TECHNIQUE 2

NOTES

....
....
....
....

Wrestling Training Log

DATE WEEKS HOURS TRAINED
COACH TIME

GOALS

WARM UP / DRILLS

TECHNIQUE 1

TECHNIQUE 2

NOTES

Wrestling Training Log

DATE   **WEEKS**   **HOURS TRAINED**

COACH   **TIME**

GOALS

WARM UP / DRILLS

TECHNIQUE 1

TECHNIQUE 2

NOTES

....
....
....
....

Wrestling Training Log

DATE   **WEEKS**   **HOURS TRAINED**

COACH   **TIME**

GOALS

WARM UP / DRILLS

TECHNIQUE 1

TECHNIQUE 2

NOTES

Wrestling Training Log

DATE　　　　　**WEEKS**　　　　　**HOURS TRAINED**
COACH　　　　　　　　　　　　　**TIME**

GOALS

WARM UP / DRILLS

TECHNIQUE 1

TECHNIQUE 2

NOTES

Wrestling Training Log

DATE　　　　**WEEKS**　　　　**HOURS TRAINED**
COACH　　　　　　　　　　　**TIME**

GOALS

WARM UP / DRILLS

TECHNIQUE 1

TECHNIQUE 2

NOTES

....
....
....
....

Wrestling Training Log

DATE **WEEKS** **HOURS TRAINED**
COACH **TIME**

GOALS

WARM UP / DRILLS

TECHNIQUE 1

TECHNIQUE 2

NOTES

....
....
....
....

Wrestling Training Log

DATE WEEKS HOURS TRAINED
COACH TIME

GOALS

WARM UP / DRILLS

TECHNIQUE 1

TECHNIQUE 2

NOTES

....
....
....
....

Wrestling Training Log

DATE **WEEKS** **HOURS TRAINED**
COACH **TIME**

GOALS

WARM UP / DRILLS

TECHNIQUE 1

TECHNIQUE 2

NOTES

Wrestling Training Log

DATE WEEKS HOURS TRAINED
COACH TIME

GOALS

WARM UP / DRILLS

TECHNIQUE 1

TECHNIQUE 2

NOTES

Wrestling Training Log

DATE   WEEKS   HOURS TRAINED
COACH   TIME

GOALS

WARM UP / DRILLS

TECHNIQUE 1

TECHNIQUE 2

NOTES

Wrestling Training Log

DATE WEEKS HOURS TRAINED
COACH TIME

GOALS

WARM UP / DRILLS

TECHNIQUE 1

TECHNIQUE 2

NOTES

Wrestling Training Log

DATE **WEEKS** **HOURS TRAINED**
COACH **TIME**

GOALS

WARM UP / DRILLS

TECHNIQUE 1

TECHNIQUE 2

NOTES

....
....
....
....

Wrestling Training Log

DATE   **WEEKS**   **HOURS TRAINED**
COACH   **TIME**

GOALS

WARM UP / DRILLS

TECHNIQUE 1

TECHNIQUE 2

NOTES

Wrestling Training Log

DATE **WEEKS** **HOURS TRAINED**
COACH **TIME**

GOALS

WARM UP / DRILLS

TECHNIQUE 1

TECHNIQUE 2

NOTES

....
....
....
....

Wrestling Training Log

DATE   **WEEKS**   **HOURS TRAINED**
COACH   **TIME**

GOALS

WARM UP / DRILLS

TECHNIQUE 1

TECHNIQUE 2

NOTES

....
....
....
....

Wrestling Training Log

DATE **WEEKS** **HOURS TRAINED**
COACH **TIME**

GOALS

WARM UP / DRILLS

TECHNIQUE 1

TECHNIQUE 2

NOTES

Wrestling Training Log

DATE WEEKS HOURS TRAINED
COACH TIME

GOALS

WARM UP / DRILLS

TECHNIQUE 1

TECHNIQUE 2

NOTES

Wrestling Training Log

DATE   WEEKS   HOURS TRAINED
COACH   TIME

GOALS

WARM UP / DRILLS

TECHNIQUE 1

TECHNIQUE 2

NOTES

....
....
....
....

Wrestling Training Log

DATE   WEEKS   HOURS TRAINED
COACH   TIME

GOALS

WARM UP / DRILLS

TECHNIQUE 1

TECHNIQUE 2

NOTES

Wrestling Training Log

DATE　　　　**WEEKS**　　　　　　**HOURS TRAINED**
COACH　　　　　　　　　　　　　**TIME**

GOALS

WARM UP / DRILLS

TECHNIQUE 1

TECHNIQUE 2

NOTES

....
....
....
....

Wrestling Training Log

DATE **WEEKS** **HOURS TRAINED**
COACH **TIME**

GOALS

WARM UP / DRILLS

TECHNIQUE 1

TECHNIQUE 2

NOTES

Wrestling Training Log

DATE　　　　　　　WEEKS　　　　　　　HOURS TRAINED

COACH　　　　　　　　　　　　　　　　TIME

GOALS

WARM UP / DRILLS

TECHNIQUE 1

TECHNIQUE 2

NOTES

....
....
....
....

Wrestling Training Log

DATE WEEKS HOURS TRAINED
COACH TIME

GOALS

WARM UP / DRILLS

TECHNIQUE 1

TECHNIQUE 2

NOTES

Wrestling Training Log

DATE **WEEKS** **HOURS TRAINED**
COACH **TIME**

GOALS

WARM UP / DRILLS

TECHNIQUE 1

TECHNIQUE 2

NOTES

....
....
....
....

Wrestling Training Log

DATE WEEKS HOURS TRAINED
COACH TIME

GOALS

WARM UP / DRILLS

TECHNIQUE 1

TECHNIQUE 2

NOTES

....
....
....
....

Wrestling Training Log

DATE　　　　　**WEEKS**　　　　　**HOURS TRAINED**
COACH　　　　　　　　　　　　　**TIME**

GOALS

WARM UP / DRILLS

TECHNIQUE 1

TECHNIQUE 2

NOTES

....
....
....
....

Wrestling Training Log

DATE　　　　　　**WEEKS**　　　　　　**HOURS TRAINED**

COACH　　　　　　　　　　　　　　　　**TIME**

GOALS

WARM UP / DRILLS

TECHNIQUE 1

TECHNIQUE 2

NOTES

....
....
....
....

Wrestling Training Log

DATE   **WEEKS**   **HOURS TRAINED**

COACH   **TIME**

GOALS

WARM UP / DRILLS

TECHNIQUE 1

TECHNIQUE 2

NOTES

Wrestling Training Log

DATE **WEEKS** **HOURS TRAINED**
COACH **TIME**

GOALS

WARM UP / DRILLS

TECHNIQUE 1

TECHNIQUE 2

NOTES

Wrestling Training Log

DATE   WEEKS   HOURS TRAINED
COACH   TIME

GOALS

WARM UP / DRILLS

TECHNIQUE 1

TECHNIQUE 2

NOTES

....
....
....
....

Wrestling Training Log

DATE　　　　**WEEKS**　　　　**HOURS TRAINED**
COACH　　　　　　　　　　　**TIME**

GOALS

WARM UP / DRILLS

TECHNIQUE 1

TECHNIQUE 2

NOTES

....
....
....
....

Wrestling Training Log

DATE **WEEKS** **HOURS TRAINED**
COACH **TIME**

GOALS

WARM UP / DRILLS

TECHNIQUE 1

TECHNIQUE 2

NOTES

Wrestling Training Log

DATE WEEKS HOURS TRAINED
COACH TIME

GOALS

WARM UP / DRILLS

TECHNIQUE 1

TECHNIQUE 2

NOTES

Wrestling Training Log

DATE **WEEKS** **HOURS TRAINED**
COACH **TIME**

GOALS

WARM UP / DRILLS

TECHNIQUE 1

TECHNIQUE 2

NOTES

Wrestling Training Log

DATE   **WEEKS**   **HOURS TRAINED**

COACH   **TIME**

GOALS

WARM UP / DRILLS

TECHNIQUE 1

TECHNIQUE 2

NOTES

Wrestling Training Log

DATE **WEEKS** **HOURS TRAINED**
COACH **TIME**

GOALS

WARM UP / DRILLS

TECHNIQUE 1

TECHNIQUE 2

NOTES

Wrestling Training Log

DATE   WEEKS   HOURS TRAINED

COACH   TIME

GOALS

WARM UP / DRILLS

TECHNIQUE 1

TECHNIQUE 2

NOTES

Wrestling Training Log

DATE **WEEKS** **HOURS TRAINED**
COACH **TIME**

GOALS

WARM UP / DRILLS

TECHNIQUE 1

TECHNIQUE 2

NOTES

Wrestling Training Log

DATE   **WEEKS**   **HOURS TRAINED**

COACH   **TIME**

GOALS

WARM UP / DRILLS

TECHNIQUE 1

TECHNIQUE 2

NOTES

Wrestling Training Log

DATE   WEEKS   HOURS TRAINED
COACH   TIME

GOALS

WARM UP / DRILLS

TECHNIQUE 1

TECHNIQUE 2

NOTES

....
....
....
....

Wrestling Training Log

DATE **WEEKS** **HOURS TRAINED**
COACH **TIME**

GOALS

WARM UP / DRILLS

TECHNIQUE 1

TECHNIQUE 2

NOTES

Wrestling Training Log

DATE   WEEKS   HOURS TRAINED
COACH   TIME

GOALS

WARM UP / DRILLS

TECHNIQUE 1

TECHNIQUE 2

NOTES

....
....
....
....

Wrestling Training Log

DATE **WEEKS** **HOURS TRAINED**
COACH **TIME**

GOALS

WARM UP / DRILLS

TECHNIQUE 1

TECHNIQUE 2

NOTES

Wrestling Training Log

DATE **WEEKS** **HOURS TRAINED**
COACH **TIME**

GOALS

WARM UP / DRILLS

TECHNIQUE 1

TECHNIQUE 2

NOTES

Wrestling Training Log

DATE **WEEKS** **HOURS TRAINED**
COACH **TIME**

GOALS

WARM UP / DRILLS

TECHNIQUE 1

TECHNIQUE 2

NOTES

Wrestling Training Log

DATE WEEKS HOURS TRAINED
COACH TIME

GOALS

WARM UP / DRILLS

TECHNIQUE 1

TECHNIQUE 2

NOTES

....
....
....
....

Wrestling Training Log

DATE   **WEEKS**   **HOURS TRAINED**

COACH   **TIME**

GOALS

WARM UP / DRILLS

TECHNIQUE 1

TECHNIQUE 2

NOTES

Wrestling Training Log

DATE **WEEKS** **HOURS TRAINED**
COACH **TIME**

GOALS

WARM UP / DRILLS

TECHNIQUE 1

TECHNIQUE 2

NOTES

Wrestling Training Log

DATE WEEKS HOURS TRAINED
COACH TIME

GOALS

WARM UP / DRILLS

TECHNIQUE 1

TECHNIQUE 2

NOTES

Wrestling Training Log

DATE   **WEEKS**   **HOURS TRAINED**

COACH   **TIME**

GOALS

WARM UP / DRILLS

TECHNIQUE 1

TECHNIQUE 2

NOTES

....
....
....
....

Wrestling Training Log

DATE **WEEKS** **HOURS TRAINED**
COACH **TIME**

GOALS

WARM UP / DRILLS

TECHNIQUE 1

TECHNIQUE 2

NOTES

Wrestling Training Log

DATE **WEEKS** **HOURS TRAINED**
COACH **TIME**

GOALS

WARM UP / DRILLS

TECHNIQUE 1

TECHNIQUE 2

NOTES

Wrestling Training Log

DATE WEEKS HOURS TRAINED
COACH TIME

GOALS

WARM UP / DRILLS

TECHNIQUE 1

TECHNIQUE 2

NOTES

....
....
....
....

Wrestling Training Log

DATE **WEEKS** **HOURS TRAINED**
COACH **TIME**

GOALS

WARM UP / DRILLS

TECHNIQUE 1

TECHNIQUE 2

NOTES

Wrestling Training Log

DATE WEEKS HOURS TRAINED
COACH TIME

GOALS

WARM UP / DRILLS

TECHNIQUE 1

TECHNIQUE 2

NOTES

Wrestling Training Log

DATE   **WEEKS**   **HOURS TRAINED**

COACH   **TIME**

GOALS

WARM UP / DRILLS

TECHNIQUE 1

TECHNIQUE 2

NOTES

....
....
....
....

Wrestling Training Log

DATE   **WEEKS**   **HOURS TRAINED**

COACH   **TIME**

GOALS

WARM UP / DRILLS

TECHNIQUE 1

TECHNIQUE 2

NOTES

....
....
....
....

Wrestling Training Log

DATE　　　　　　　WEEKS　　　　　　　HOURS TRAINED
COACH　　　　　　　　　　　　　　　　TIME

GOALS

WARM UP / DRILLS

TECHNIQUE 1

TECHNIQUE 2

NOTES

Wrestling Training Log

DATE   WEEKS   HOURS TRAINED

COACH   TIME

GOALS

WARM UP / DRILLS

TECHNIQUE 1

TECHNIQUE 2

NOTES

Wrestling Training Log

DATE   **WEEKS**   **HOURS TRAINED**

COACH   **TIME**

GOALS

WARM UP / DRILLS

TECHNIQUE 1

TECHNIQUE 2

NOTES

....
....
....
....

Wrestling Training Log

DATE   **WEEKS**   **HOURS TRAINED**
COACH   **TIME**

GOALS

WARM UP / DRILLS

TECHNIQUE 1

TECHNIQUE 2

NOTES

Wrestling Training Log

DATE **WEEKS** **HOURS TRAINED**
COACH **TIME**

GOALS

WARM UP / DRILLS

TECHNIQUE 1

TECHNIQUE 2

NOTES

....
....
....
....

Wrestling Training Log

DATE   **WEEKS**   **HOURS TRAINED**

COACH   **TIME**

GOALS

WARM UP / DRILLS

TECHNIQUE 1

TECHNIQUE 2

NOTES

....
....
....
....

Wrestling Training Log

DATE WEEKS HOURS TRAINED
COACH TIME

GOALS

WARM UP / DRILLS

TECHNIQUE 1

TECHNIQUE 2

NOTES

....
....
....
....

Wrestling Training Log

DATE **WEEKS** **HOURS TRAINED**

COACH **TIME**

GOALS

WARM UP / DRILLS

TECHNIQUE 1

TECHNIQUE 2

NOTES

Wrestling Training Log

DATE　　　　　**WEEKS**　　　　　**HOURS TRAINED**
COACH　　　　　　　　　　　　　**TIME**

GOALS

WARM UP / DRILLS

TECHNIQUE 1

TECHNIQUE 2

NOTES

....
....
....
....

Wrestling Training Log

DATE　　　　**WEEKS**　　　　**HOURS TRAINED**
COACH　　　　　　　　　　　**TIME**

GOALS

WARM UP / DRILLS

TECHNIQUE 1

TECHNIQUE 2

NOTES

....
....
....
....

Wrestling Training Log

DATE　　　　　**WEEKS**　　　　　**HOURS TRAINED**

COACH　　　　　　　　　　　　　**TIME**

GOALS

WARM UP / DRILLS

TECHNIQUE 1

TECHNIQUE 2

NOTES

....
....
....
....

Wrestling Training Log

DATE   **WEEKS**   **HOURS TRAINED**

COACH   **TIME**

GOALS

WARM UP / DRILLS

TECHNIQUE 1

TECHNIQUE 2

NOTES

Wrestling Training Log

DATE **WEEKS** **HOURS TRAINED**
COACH **TIME**

GOALS

WARM UP / DRILLS

TECHNIQUE 1

TECHNIQUE 2

NOTES

Wrestling Training Log

DATE **WEEKS** **HOURS TRAINED**
COACH **TIME**

GOALS

WARM UP / DRILLS

TECHNIQUE 1

TECHNIQUE 2

NOTES

Wrestling Training Log

DATE　　　　　　　WEEKS　　　　　　　HOURS TRAINED

COACH　　　　　　　　　　　　　　　　TIME

GOALS

WARM UP / DRILLS

TECHNIQUE 1

TECHNIQUE 2

NOTES

Wrestling Training Log

DATE   **WEEKS**   **HOURS TRAINED**

COACH   **TIME**

GOALS

WARM UP / DRILLS

TECHNIQUE 1

TECHNIQUE 2

NOTES

Wrestling Training Log

DATE **WEEKS** **HOURS TRAINED**
COACH **TIME**

GOALS

WARM UP / DRILLS

TECHNIQUE 1

TECHNIQUE 2

NOTES

Wrestling Training Log

DATE WEEKS HOURS TRAINED
COACH TIME

GOALS

WARM UP / DRILLS

TECHNIQUE 1

TECHNIQUE 2

NOTES

Wrestling Training Log

DATE WEEKS HOURS TRAINED
COACH TIME

GOALS

WARM UP / DRILLS

TECHNIQUE 1

TECHNIQUE 2

NOTES

Wrestling Training Log

DATE WEEKS HOURS TRAINED
COACH TIME

GOALS

WARM UP / DRILLS

TECHNIQUE 1

TECHNIQUE 2

NOTES

Wrestling Training Log

DATE **WEEKS** **HOURS TRAINED**
COACH **TIME**

GOALS

WARM UP / DRILLS

TECHNIQUE 1

TECHNIQUE 2

NOTES
....
....
....
....

Wrestling Training Log

DATE	WEEKS	HOURS TRAINED
COACH	 	TIME

GOALS

WARM UP / DRILLS

TECHNIQUE 1

TECHNIQUE 2

NOTES

Wrestling Training Log

DATE **WEEKS** **HOURS TRAINED**
COACH **TIME**

GOALS

WARM UP / DRILLS

TECHNIQUE 1

TECHNIQUE 2

NOTES

....
....
....
....

Wrestling Training Log

DATE　　　　　　　WEEKS　　　　　　　HOURS TRAINED
COACH　　　　　　　　　　　　　　　　TIME

GOALS

WARM UP / DRILLS

TECHNIQUE 1

TECHNIQUE 2

NOTES

....
....
....
....

Wrestling Training Log

DATE **WEEKS** **HOURS TRAINED**
COACH **TIME**

GOALS

WARM UP / DRILLS

TECHNIQUE 1

TECHNIQUE 2

NOTES

www.ingramcontent.com/pod-product-compliance
Lightning Source LLC
Chambersburg PA
CBHW071406080526
44587CB00017B/3191